I0421070

Post-Action Strategic Debriefing©

Procedural workbook
and integrated leader's guide.

Amy S. Morgan, MSC

Post-Action Strategic Debriefing©

Procedural workbook
and integrated leader's guide.

First Edition

•

AMY S. MORGAN, MSC

Copyright © 2015 Amy S. Morgan, MSC
All rights reserved.
No part of this publication may be reproduced or transmitted
in any form or by any means, electronic, mechanical, photocopying,
recording, or otherwise without the prior permission of the author.

This book may be purchased at a reduced price, in bulk quantities,
by contacting the author.

ISBN-13: 978-1517013462
ISBN-10: 1517013461

Author contact information:

Amy S. Morgan, MSC
Email: AmySMorgan@yahoo.com
405-219-0291

Post-Action Strategic Debriefing©

Summary

In the line of duty, whether it is public-safety or another industry, there will be the inevitable critical incident on the job, which can result at times in physical injury or even fatality. The incident may also create another type of injury, more difficult to detect but often lasting much longer than a physical injury, and one that can cause safety issues in the future. Post-Action Strategic Debriefing© addresses the incident immediately after, using a technique of combined aspects of critical incident stress debriefing and the after-action review, as well as counseling and intervention methods. Those involved in the incident go through a guided process of reviewing the intended plan, the reality of the incident, actions to reinforce in the future and those that can be used as opportunities for positive change,. The PASD© process also focuses on preventing ongoing trauma effects from the incident as well as creating a positive momentum for the team to be stronger, more united, and more mentally healthy following the incident. The PASD© process is designed to be performed after each type of incident, with a leader's guide integrated into a step-by-step workbook format for the group to follow.

DISCLAIMER:

The Post-Action Strategic Debriefing© process is the result of a combination of aspects from multiple post-incident techniques. The PASD© process is a strategic mental-wellness focused process designed to assist team leaders start the conversations within their team that may lead to team members seeking further resources for more in-depth and long-term help. It does not constitute the equivalent of a certified debriefing session, licensed counseling, or any type of therapeutic intervention. It is a starting point for discussion. The author is not responsible for individual or team outcomes or mental health issues resulting from any incidents or the PASD© session(s), as those are unattended by the author. It is recommended that team leaders and individuals seek long-term help through available local resources for any mental health illnesses or disorders resulting from a critical incident.

For a full database of your local mental health resources, please call 2-1-1.

For thoughts of suicide, please call 800-273-8255 (TALK) immediately.

TABLE OF CONTENTS

Post-Action Strategic Debriefing©

Why

1
Being Mentally
& Emotionally Healthy

Most people understand what it means to be physically healthy. Generally one has good heart, lung, and other-organ health, mobility, and can function with all or most body parts working the way they were intended to work. Mental health follows the same guidelines, but deals with mental capacity and the brain's ability to function well. If one is able to think fairly clearly, cope with regular life situations, including stressors and challenges, be flexible with one's thinking, and solve basic problems by thinking of viable solutions, then he/she is probably considered to be in a good state of mental health. Based on these guidelines, then, we can understand the meaning of emotional health. If an individual is able to function well emotionally, this means they are in good control of their emotions, and also the behavior that frequently accompanies emotions. If a life challenge arises, an emotionally healthy person will manage his emotions through the challenge, and will then have some resilience and bounce back to his normal emotional level pretty quickly after the challenge is resolved.

It is widely believed that physical, emotional, and mental health are all closely related and each affects the other.   For example, if one has a chronic physical disease, like cancer, this can have a tremendous impact on one's emotional health, causing depression or anxiety. Physical illness that is ongoing (chronic) or even diagnosed as terminal can have the greatest negative effect because it produces a sense of hopelessness, but also causes mental and emotional fatigue in the individual dealing with the chronic pain or illness. We will discuss fatigue in more detail in chapter five. Conversely, mental illness or disorders can also affect one's emotional health, decreasing the ability to control emotions and potentially the behaviors that correspond to the emotions. For example, if an individual is coping with a significant amount of stress, or an addiction, this can directly impact his emotional health – irritability or sadness - as well as his physical health -ulcers are frequently caused by high stress levels.

Taking continuous care of all three – physical, emotional, and mental health -- can create in an individual a better preparedness and level of resiliency for stressful events or injuries. Exercise and an ongoing physical fitness routine create a stronger physical body that can more easily recover from an illness or injury. Likewise, ongoing and continual mental exercise strengthens one's ability toward problem-solving, adapting to change, building and maintaining successful relationships, and functioning in social environments.

How does one strengthen mental and emotional health? It's important to try to achieve a balance, by lowering stress and increasing positive activities. Participating in positive activities like exercise, fun, hobbies, doing good deeds for others, taking the time to enjoy family and friends, and just positive thinking overall. Positive activities like these can release endorphins, aiding one's ability to feel less pain, and to have controlled emotions. Endorphins are chemicals that originate in different parts of the body like the brain and nervous system, the spinal cord, and the pituitary gland. They work as neurotransmitters, connecting to the opioid receptors in the brain that are mostly responsible for blocking pain and controlling emotion. These endorphins are naturally created by the body and work just like a narcotic such as heroin or morphine. The endorphins in the body are able to block pain, but also create feelings of pleasure. Endorphins are designed to regulate themselves, so that one does not engage in too much pleasure which could actually cause harm, but also to create enough to keep an individual from things like rage or anxiety.

It is believed that our neurotransmitters can be "trained" to connect better, helping us to be stronger emotionally, just like bodies can be trained physically to function better. The theory is that if one is depressed, emotionally imbalanced, negative, etc., the neurotransmitters are not connecting properly. Picture a spark between two items that just isn't connecting – the spark misses the second item and never connects the two. This is how neuro transmitters work, sort of – when one is thinking positively and functioning with good mental and emotional health, the neurotransmitters are connecting. The training of these connections then is by purposely making the neurotransmitters connect, training them to then do this on their own. The more positive thoughts one focuses on, whether reading them, repeating them, or just continuously focusing on positives all day long, the more often the neurotransmitters are connecting. The more they connect, the more they learn to naturally connect.

The more endorphins released, and the better your neurotransmitters are connecting, the more mentally and emotionally healthy the individual. Not having good, strong emotional and mental health can affect an individual by making them more prone to illness, more susceptible to emotional outbursts of anger, fear, irritability, etc. It can also lead to substance abuse, hopelessness, and a disintegration of relationships, jobs, and the ability to function normally in society. By strengthening the emotional and mental health, one becomes more resilient and better able to cope with stressors that arise. This makes for less unpredictability, better focus, and on the job, fewer accidents.

2
Trauma

Trauma is a word that is frequently used generically in a wide variety of situations, intended to describe something scary or maybe upsetting. The most basic and pointed definition of trauma is that it is an emotional response to an extremely unpleasant experience. In many cases, the extremely unpleasant experience also has the 'shock factor' of being an unexpected experience; but this does not have to be true in order for an experience to cause trauma.

Incidents like intentional violence or being a witness to it, violations of acceptable 'normal' societal behavior like war, torture, rape, etc., and even particular 'everyday' events like divorce, poverty, or discrimination can be seen as traumatic events. It is largely based on the perception of the individual experiencing the incident that determines whether it is traumatic or not. However, for the most part, incidents that cause trauma are generally accepted as distressing, by the majority.

It is important during the Post-Action Strategic Debriefing© process to communicate to all participants that trauma is a normal emotional response to an extremely unpleasant experience. For those in the group who have more difficulty admitting that any experience or incident may have upset them in any way, it might be helpful to remind the entire group that the traumatic response is the normal response to this type of incident. The abnormal response would be to feel nothing, or to have no reaction – individuals who have no sense of ethics or the rights of other people, who feel no empathy and who are callous to the concern of the feelings of others, who have an inability to feel emotions deeply, and who have a very high tolerance for what others might consider 'repulsive' are diagnosed as sociopaths or psychopaths. Sharing this factual bit of information with the group might actually give permission to those who want to appear tough and strong to allow themselves to acknowledge and speak about the emotional responses they are experiencing. A leader will essentially be reiterating here that it is normal and acceptable to have emotions related to a critical incident.

On the job, depending on the industry, there are many different potential incidents which are considered critical and potentially trauma-causing. The Post-Action Strategic Debriefing© process is designed to alleviate the effects of an incident on one's trauma responses. Meaning, in short, by using the PASD© process, the goal is for those involved to leave the room with a sense of healing after the incident, as well as an emotional and mental strength and resilience to move forward without lasting negative effects of trauma. The PASD© process, though, is a starting point and a process for being a catalyst for discussion and openness that might not otherwise be facilitated. Trauma has many potential long-term effects, and those involved in a traumatic incident would most likely benefit from seeking long-term mental health resources for all the trauma responses that may occur over time following the incident.

3
Prevention / Preparedness

As mentioned previously, being of strong mental and emotional health makes one resilient to future stressors. The best way to bounce back from a traumatic experience is to first be as prepared as possible – physically, mentally, and emotionally. An individual who is already 'down', whether just in mood and an overall feeling of hopelessness, or whether going through an actual state of depression, or if dealing with a chronic mental health disorder or disability, the ability to manage a new stressor will be diminished. This individual is already somewhat depleted in mental and emotional strength, and will therefore not manage or respond to new stressors as well as someone who is mentally and emotionally healthy.

How does a team leader, then, train the team members to be in the best position for prevention, and be best prepared for a potential critical incident? Training is the answer – physical training for physical health, mental and emotional training, for an overall holistic state of health and well-being. Keeping team members mentally and emotionally healthy can be done through several methods:

- Develop coping skills by practicing the response procedure for potential future incidents.
- Use meditation and relaxation techniques like deep breathing, focus exercises using 'positive thoughts' training for neurotransmitters.
- Maintain a balance between work, family, fun, and downtime.
- Get enough sleep. Sleep greatly affects one's ability to respond in a healthy manner.
- Develop friendships and social relationships – by having friendships and social support network like family, church, community, teams, etc., one has more resiliency and strength because of his sense of support.
- Laugh and have fun. Humor can play a positive role in one's mental and emotional health.
- Spend some spiritual time. Spirituality, whether it be the belief in one higher power, or an overall focus on life purpose and a sense of well-being, can have many health benefits.
- Eat healthy. Nutrition – the better nutrients one's body gets, the better it is able to function in every capacity.

Strengthening one's ability to be mentally/emotionally flexible, to be able to cope with change, to see alternatives and solutions to a problem, to be resourceful, and to mentally persevere through challenges will help an individual to be better prepared should an incident occur. By being better prepared, the incident will seem less traumatic and will have fewer residual effects.

4
Post-Traumatic Stress Disorder

The American Psychiatric Association, in the Diagnostic and Statistical Manual of Mental Disorders, Fifth edition, provides a very detailed list of criteria for diagnosing Posttraumatic Stress Disorder (PTSD), summarized for brevity here:

1. Exposure to actual or threatened death, serious injury, or sexual violence in one (or more) of the following ways: Direct experience, witnessing the event as it occurred to others, learning that the event occurred to a close family member or friend, experiencing repeated or extreme exposure to aversive details of the

traumatic event (first responders collecting human remains, police officers repeatedly exposed to details of child abuse).

2. Presence of one (or more) of the following intrusion symptoms associated with the traumatic event(s), beginning after the event occurred: Recurrent, involuntary, and intrusive distressing memories of the traumatic event, recurrent distressing dreams in which the content and/or affect of the dream are related to the traumatic event; dissociative reactions (e.g. flashbacks) in which the individual feels or acts as if the traumatic event(s) were recurring, intense or prolonged psychological distress at exposure to internal or external cues that symbolize or resemble an aspect of the traumatic event(s), and marked physiological reactions to internal or external cues that symbolize or resemble an aspect of the traumatic event(s).

3. Persistent avoidance of stimuli associated with the traumatic event(s), beginning after the traumatic event(s) occurred, as evidenced by one or both of the following: Avoidance of or efforts to avoid distressing memories, thoughts, or feelings about or closely associated with the traumatic event(s), and avoidance of or efforts to avoid external reminders (people, places, conversations, activities, objects, situations) that arouse distressing memories, thoughts, or feelings about or closely associated with the traumatic event(s).

4. Negative alterations in cognitions and mood associated with the traumatic event(s), beginning or worsening after the traumatic event(s) occurred, as evidenced by two (or more) of the following: Inability to remember an important aspect of the traumatic event(s), persistent and exaggerated negative beliefs or expectations about oneself, others, or the word, persistent, distorted cognitions about the cause or consequences of the traumatic event(s) that lead the individual to blame himself/herself or others, persistent negative emotional state, markedly diminished interest or participation in significant activities, feelings of detachment or estrangement from others, persistent inability to experience positive emotions.

5. Marked alterations in arousal and reactivity associated with the traumatic event(s), beginning or worsening after the traumatic event(s) occurred, as evidenced by two (or more) of the following: Irritable behavior and angry

outbursts (with little or no provocation) typically expressed as verbal or physical aggression toward people or objects, reckless or self-destructive behavior, hypervigilance, exaggerated startle response, problems with concentration, sleep disturbance; duration of the disturbance is more than 1 month; The disturbance causes clinically significant distress or impairment in social, occupational, or other important areas of functioning; the disturbance is not attributable to the physiological effects of a substance.

This information is provided as a brief generalization of PTSD; the DSM-V should be reviewed for full details and explanation of this disorder and its effects.

A critical incident can be traumatic, and that trauma can greatly damage one's state of emotional health and well-being. The PASD© process, or any post-action, post-incident review, debriefing, or defusing process can help with immediate and short-term management of the emotions caused by the incident. However, it is not proven that the process/session alone will prevent PTSD. Long-term care such as counseling is recommended to fully avoid posttraumatic stress disorder. This is particularly true for an individual who already has PTSD and then experiences a new traumatic experience, because compounded traumatic events in one's life can have a debilitating effect on the mental and emotional health that can last a lifetime.

5
Mental/Emotional Fatigue

Mental/emotional fatigue is addressed here because it can be both a cause and a symptom of poor health. Particularly in public service careers, this fatigue comes from giving of oneself for an altruistic cause or purpose, and is sometimes called, "compassion fatigue." Essentially, those who help others tend to grow weary from giving of themselves and not taking care of themselves equally. Also, those with chronic pain or illness can grow weary from their suffering, which takes a toll on their mental and emotional strength and well-being.

The term 'depletion' is one of the ways to describe this state. When dealing with excessive and ongoing demands, stress, illness, or exhaustion, one's ability to cope and be resilient or bounce back from a stressor becomes weakened. Someone who is in this state of mental/emotional fatigue is not going to be able to respond as quickly to, or recover from, an emergency situation. On the job, this may put the individual and/or his team members at risk. The longer one remains in this state, the more depleted and unable to cope he becomes.

Example: If you hold out your hand, palm up, and someone places a book on your hand and asks you to carry it around for them, you may have no trouble at all, for a long while, carrying that book for them. If someone else then comes to you and places another book on top, and asks you to carry it also, you can do that for some time. However, the more books that are placed on you (representing the needs and demands of others, or representing stressors, pressures, difficult circumstances, negative events, etc.), the more difficult it is to carry those books on your hand. You may be able to carry those 'stressors' for a short period of time, but the longer you're carrying them around, the more difficult the task becomes. Consider carrying these for quite a while, and imagine the pain starting to increase in your hand and arm, possibly your back, from the ongoing weight. At first you may have been able to focus on everything going on around you while you were holding the one book, and even a few, but little by little as new books are added, your only area of focus becomes the books on your hand, the weight, the discomfort and pain, and your desire to drop the books. You are no longer able to focus on what's going on around you, and really could reach the point where nothing around you matters except for the pain you are experiencing. Your ability to respond to other things, to be aware and prepared for other things, and to give of yourself to anything outside of carrying those books becomes depleted.

The example above is one way to describe how someone may feel if he or she is not mentally and emotionally strong and healthy due to too many pressures or stressors, too much pain (emotional, physical), or from having not healed from an experience. Having someone in this situation on the job will put others at risk, as well as the individual, because of being unprepared and ill-equipped to fully respond to unexpected circumstances. If a critical incident were to occur with this individual on the scene, he/she will most likely not have the proper tools available mentally to be resourceful, to think quickly about alternative solutions, to persevere, and/or to guide others to safety. The more mentally and emotionally healthy team members are, the stronger the team, the more quickly the team will be able to respond in an emergency situation, the better they will be able to work together, and the fewer the safety risks that will be present.

Keeping individuals on a team, as well as the team unit itself, healthy is to strengthen the potential of a team when it comes to an incident occurring. The better an incident is handled by emotionally, mentally and physically healthy team members the better the team will bounce back and be able to move forward productively.

6
Good Health Leads to Safety

Just like being physically strong can help fend off an attacker, being healthy overall (physically, mentally, emotionally) can help safeguard against the effects of most unexpected and offensive intrusions into daily routine. Good overall health leads to resiliency and immunity against common attackers like stress, but also helps to prepare for the unexpected or emergency interference like that of a critical incident or event.

If a team is all well-balanced emotionally, mentally and physically and a critical incident event occurs, they are going to much better manage that event than if they are highly stressed, weary, depressed, or otherwise mentally/emotionally less than fully healthy. A healthy brain will be able to think creatively, quickly, and outside the normal parameters of a situation to find a solution and to be flexible with options. An emotionally or mentally depleted individual will have fewer resources available to him when the time of an emergency arises. Keeping healthy in all areas only benefits the individual, the team, and the future safety of all, should an incident arise.

Post-Action Strategic Debriefing©

What

7
Foundational Techniques

Post-Action Strategic Debriefing© is based on some aspects of the widely accepted and utilized method of critical incident stress debriefing, as well as the military's after-action review, but also combines counseling theory and techniques as well as intervention methods. This process, then, is one start to finish, step-by-step method of reviewing an incident or event by looking at what was expected to happen, what really did happen, how the team managed the incident as far as what worked and what could be improved upon in future situations, and how the team members are responding to the incident. The process looks at individual perceptions as well as team perceptions, and uses those to develop a move-forward action plan so that the team leaves the incident with a unified perspective and common understanding of what happened and how it may affect them as a team and individually. The PASD© process also includes an aspect of resource recommendation for longer term management of the emotions, thoughts and feelings the team members may take away from the experience of the incident.

Post-Action Strategic Debriefing©

HOW

8
The Process Outline

The Post-Action Strategic Debriefing© process follows five main steps. These five steps are explained in detail, with instructions for the team leader to use with the team, in the following sections.

1. Gather Together

2. Expectations vs. Reality

3. Positive Reframing

4. Getting Back to Center

5. Follow-Up Plan

Post-Action Strategic Debriefing©

Use the
Post-Action Strategic Debriefing©
Process

Leader: This workbook is designed to be used by you, the leader, to walk your team through this process step by step. It is recommended that notes be taken in the workbook and that a new workbook be used for each separate incident. It is, though, up to you what or how much you document. Your specific situation may be of a confidential or secure nature that permits you only to write down very basic information, with little or no documentation desired. Or, you may want to use this as your full documentation resource for each incident and keep these as part of your historical incident records.

Post-Action Strategic Debriefing©

Step One
Gather Together

The more quickly after an incident the team can gather together, the more effective this process will be. Immediately following (within 1-3 hours) is recommended because 1) most of those individuals involved in the incident are still in the location or vicinity and can more easily participate; 2) those involved will have heightened emotions during this time period and therefore may be more willing to share their emotions; and 3) memories are more clear, often, immediately after an incident. However, you may encourage participants to bring forward any additional thoughts, emotions or memories they have after the PASD© session is completed. If the 1-3 hour time frame is not possible, attempt to complete the PASD© session at least within 24 hours after the incident.

If you'd like, list the names of those involved in the incident here, and note whether they are attending the session or not:

Name   Yes   No

_____   _____   _____

_____   _____   _____

_____   _____   _____

_____   _____   _____

_____   _____   _____

_____   _____   _____

_____   _____   _____

_____   _____   _____

_____   _____   _____

_____   _____   _____

_____   _____   _____

_____   _____   _____

Leader, read this to the team:

In this room, there are no rankings or hierarchy when it comes to speaking – this is an all-are-equal venue for recounting the details of the incident from all perspectives, understanding and respecting that each individual person has their own perspective of the incident. There is to be no blame placed, and all events should be recalled as fact only, remembering that during this process all perspectives are equal and what may appear as fault from one perspective may appear quite differently from another.

We are gathered here as a team, and we remain a team throughout. A team member who is speaking is not to be interrupted, and we are all here to encourage each other, to remain strong together, and to remember that we all went through this experience together. We will discuss it, gain strength from it, and we will leave this room as a stronger, more cohesive team because of our experience.

1.   Please breathe in and out, slowly and deeply, to help yourselves become more physically able to speak, to listen, to focus, and to be productive during this session. If you become anxious at any part of this session, remember this deep, slow breathing technique and repeat it as often as necessary. We have just experienced something distressing, and it is completely normal for our anxiety level to be high right now; so taking the effort to breathe slowly will physiologically reduce that anxiety.

2.   Please know and understand that you have just experienced a traumatic event. Trauma is an emotional response to an extremely unpleasant, and often an unexpected, experience. To walk away with no emotional affect is the most uncommon response; to be here, right now, experiencing possibly chaotic thoughts and emotions, is the very normal response.

3.   We are going to share our perspectives of this experience without judgment on each other or ourselves, and acknowledge that emotions are a normal reaction, and those are completely acceptable in this session because they will make us a stronger, more cohesive team with members who know and understand each other better.

Post-Action Strategic Debriefing©

Step Two
Expectations vs. Reality

Leader, facilitate the team's answering of these questions. If you prefer, ask for volunteer responses and take those from whoever is willing to participate. This process should be voluntary. If you prefer to go around the room, asking each person individually, that will work but keep in mind that no one should be forced to share if for some reason they are unwilling. These individuals, though, may need to be addressed later and offered resources or help if their reasons for not participating may have to do with shock or severe trauma from the experience.

1.   What was our mission and/or our goal (what was supposed to happen)? (Leader: This particularly applies if your team was sent in on a mission and is now reflecting back on the way that mission went or was handled. If this session is due to an unexpected emergency situation, reflect on whether your team was, or was not, prepared, and what those preparations (or lack of) for this type of incident were.)

_____

_____

_____

_____

_____

_____

_____

_____

_____

_____

_____

_____

_____

_____

_____

_____

_____

_____

_____

If you need more space, please add additional paper to your documentation.

2.   What actually happened (this is where different perspectives will be
revealed)? – encourage brief answers in this section.

_____

_____

_____

_____

_____

_____

_____

_____

_____

_____

_____

_____

_____

_____

_____

_____

_____

_____

If you need more space, please add additional paper to your documentation.

3.   What worked well, that we would want to repeat in the future in other similar crisis, emergency, or critical incident type situations?

_____

_____

_____

_____

_____

_____

_____

_____

_____

_____

_____

_____

_____

_____

_____

_____

_____

_____

_____

_____

_____

_____

_____

_____

_____

_____

_____

_____

_____

_____

_____

_____

_____

_____

_____

_____

If you need more space, please add additional paper to your documentation.

4.   What challenges did we encounter, what could be improved, and what areas were our team's areas of weakness and need for growth? These are the areas we can use as opportunities to become stronger, more fit, and more prepared for future incidents:

_____

_____

_____

_____

_____

_____

_____

_____

_____

_____

_____

_____

_____

_____

_____

_____

_____

_____

_____

_____

_____

_____

_____

_____

_____

_____

_____

_____

_____

_____

_____

_____

_____

_____

_____

_____

If you need more space, please add additional paper to your documentation.

5. What are your thoughts on the experience we have just been through? (Ask each member to provide one first and foremost thought that entered their mind when the incident occurred.)

_____

_____

_____

_____

_____

_____

_____

_____

_____

_____

_____

_____

_____

_____

_____

_____

_____

_____

_____

_____

_____

_____

_____

_____

_____

_____

_____

_____

_____

_____

_____

_____

_____

_____

_____

_____

_____

If you need more space, please add additional paper to your documentation.

6.   What reactions did this incident bring forward for you? (You might encourage answers to this question by asking what they felt was the worst part or most difficult to experience of this incident.)

_____

_____

_____

_____

_____

_____

_____

_____

_____

_____

_____

_____

_____

_____

_____

_____

_____

_____

_____

_____

_____

_____

_____

_____

_____

_____

_____

_____

_____

_____

_____

_____

_____

_____

_____

_____

_____

_____

_____

_____

_____

If you need more space, please add additional paper to your documentation.

7. How do you think this incident might have an effect on you after you leave this room today? (Allow each participant to answer with a 1-2 sentence response to this question.)

_____

_____

_____

_____

_____

_____

_____

_____

_____

_____

_____

_____

_____

_____

_____

_____

_____

_____

_____

_____

_____

_____

_____

_____

_____

_____

_____

_____

_____

_____

_____

_____

_____

_____

_____

_____

_____

_____

_____

If you need more space, please add additional paper to your documentation.

Post-Action Strategic Debriefing©

Step Three
Positive Reframing

Team members may be experiencing a huge variety of emotions and thoughts related to the incident. They will, most likely, lean toward the negative and the danger and/or potential loss that was associated with the incident.

One way team members can come back together and turn the negative incident into a learning or growing experience is to try and reframe the "what happened" responses into more positive perspectives. The facts do not change, but the emotions related to them become less harmful.

An example of reframing would be: A husband, wife and their 2 children are in a car, with the husband driving. The children are being a little rowdy, the wife/mom is getting a little stressed, and the husband is trying to focus on his driving while also trying to help with the kids. The husband turns around to look at the kids, and this results in them running a red light and being struck by an oncoming vehicle, and all four of them being hospitalized. The wife may tell her perspective story by saying the kids were stressing her out, the husband was not paying attention to his driving because he's a bad driver, and then her stress level was already high, and the situation and his bad driving just made it worse.

The facts remain the same, once she tells the story, but the wife may choose to reframe it into a more positive perspective by changing only one element of her perspective – she may, instead, say that the kids were being loud, she was stressed, and because her husband cares about her happiness/stress level, and wants to also be a good, involved, father, he turned around to help with the kids, causing them to accidentally hit another car.

This takes away blame, which also will then remove/reduce anger and/or resentment which could potentially cause long-term damage to the marriage relationship and the family (team).

Reframing, again, one step further, could also change the kids' obnoxious behavior (because it could be seen later as a cause for the wreck, which would then also cause anger/resentment) in this way: The kids were very excited about their destination, and, because they are kids, they were not containing their excitement level or emotions, which resulted in them being louder than normal. Mom was excited for them but trying to manage their noise level so that they didn't distract their dad, who was driving the car. This takes away the blame from the children, and shows them as just acting in a way that is normal and acceptable for their age and the situation.

By reframing this entire story, the facts remain intact, but blame and anger are removed, and all parties are seen as equally having gone through the same situation together, none of them being to blame, and all of them being distressed by the outcome, together.

Use brief examples of the facts initially provided in the "what happened" section, and ask team members to reframe, removing blame or just providing a more positive, or even more neutral, perspective on the detail of the incident.

_____

_____

_____

_____

_____

_____

_____

_____

_____

_____

_____

_____

_____

_____

_____

_____

_____

_____

_____

If you need more space, please add additional paper to your documentation.

Step Four
Getting Back to Center

It is frequently said that, after something traumatic happens, one never feels 'normal' again, but that the individual will start to live with a 'new normal'. This acknowledges that something traumatic happened, and does not attempt to pretend it did not, but also moves the individual toward still having hope of a sense of normalcy, stability, and strong emotional and mental health.

To bring the individuals in this team back together, to form a stronger and more cohesive team, in addition to stronger individuals, any anger and blame must be reduced or eliminated. By sharing together that they've all been through something traumatic as a team, a bonding experience and a sense of unity are developed.

Ask the team to list ways in which they feel this experience may help them to be a stronger team. If team members list challenges, or ways that this might actually weaken their team, ask them to then brainstorm and offer solutions and discuss those, for using those challenges to help them become the stronger team. This discussion brings to the forefront any obstacles to team cohesion, but also then reiterates and encourages the team to continue thinking as a team, but also helps them to focus on using negative experiences to become stronger and to be more unified going forward.

_____

_____

_____

_____

_____

_____

_____

_____

_____

_____

_____

_____

_____

_____

_____

_____

_____

_____

If you need more space, please add additional paper to your documentation.

Post-Action Strategic Debriefing©

Step Five
Follow-Up Plan

Leader, read: These types of incidents can cause long-term mental or emotional effects on those who experience them. Please personally think of one or two people you could go to if you felt you needed to discuss your reactions to this incident after you leave here today.

Leader, then ask the group – what are some other resources that are available that might be helpful if you experience any sort of reaction to this incident and feel like it might benefit you to talk it out? Examples are:

1.   Counselor

2.   Clergy / pastor

3.   Family members / spouse

4.   Close friend

5.   Other team members

6.   Suicide talk-line (800-273-8255)

7.   _____

8.   _____

9.   _____

10.   _____

11.   _____

12.   _____

13.   _____

14.   _____

15.   _____

Remind the team that the more they are willing to use resources, the stronger they will end up being as an individual as well as a team member. Mental and emotional wellness and strength are just as important as physical health and strength, and can be trained and prepared for in the same way. Seeking mental health resources after this type of incident should be viewed the same as an individual going to the doctor or hospital after being physically injured.

This session and this process are a starting point for discussion. Please seek whatever resources and assistance you may feel you need at any point in the future. PTSD will not be prevented by this session alone.

It is helpful to have each team member, prior to dismissing the group, say aloud one positive thing about the team unit as a whole. If they want to acknowledge one particular individual, they should do so as "the team" having done the positive thing. For example, Jim was resourceful and suggested the team use a large item to block a door – say instead, "The team was resourceful in using the item…"

--End of Session--

Post-Action Strategic Debriefing©

REFERENCES

American Psychiatric Association. (2013). Trauma- and Stressor-Related Disorders. In *Diagnostic and statistical manual of mental disorders* (Fifth ed.). Arlington, VA: American Psychiatric Publishing.

CISM International. (n.d.). http://www.criticalincidentstress.com/what_is_cism_

Critical Incident Stress Management. (n.d.). Retrieved August 22, 2015, from https://en.wikipedia.org/wiki/Critical_incident_stress_management

Davis, J. A. (1998). Providing Critical Incident Stress Debriefing (CISD) to Individuals and Communities in Situational Crisis. Retrieved from http://www.aaets.org/article54.htm

Davis, J. A. (2013, February 12, 2013). Critical Incident Stress Debriefing From a Traumatic Event. *Psychology Today*. Retrieved from https://www.psychologytoday.com/blog/crimes-and-misdemeanors/201302/critical-incident-stress-debriefing-traumatic-event

Hirstein, W. (2013). What is a psychopath? Retrieved from https://www.psychologytoday.com/blog/mindmelding/201301/what-is-psychopath-0

Mcnally, R. J. (2004, April 1, 2004). Psychological debriefing doe snot prevent posttrumatic stress disorder. *Psychiatric Times*. Retrieved from http://www.psychiatrictimes.com/ptsd/psychological-debriefing-does-not-prevent-posttraumatic-stress-disorder-0

Mitchell, J. T. (n.d.). *Crisis intervention and critical incident stress management: A defense of the field*. Retrieved from http://www.icisf.org/wp-content/uploads/2013/04/Crisis-Intervention-and-Critical-Incident-Stress-Management-a-defense-of-the-field.pdf

Mitchell, J. T. (n.d.). *Critical Incident Stress Debriefing (CISD)*. Retrieved from Info Trauma website: http://www.info-trauma.org/flash/media-e/mitchellCriticalIncidentStressDebriefing.pdf

Scheve, T. (n.d.). What are endorphins? Retrieved August 23, 2015, from http://science.howstuffworks.com/life/endorphins.htm

Strategies for good mental health wellness. (n.d.). Retrieved from http://www.mhww.org/strategies.html

www.ingramcontent.com/pod-product-compliance
Lightning Source LLC
Chambersburg PA
CBHW080436290526
45791CB00008BA/2525